Yes, I Can Get Pregnant: Letters For Infertility Patients To Send
Themselves

Other Books by the Author:

Dancing Your Way to Fertility
The Infertility Diaries
Your Daily Fertility Success Journal
Super Sperm Your Guy and Beat Infertility So He Can Get You Pregnant:
The Ultimate Male Fertility Preparation Program

Visit www.dancingyourwaytofertility.com to learn more!

Yes, I Can Get Pregnant Letters For Infertility Patients To Send Themselves
Paula Fuoco Davis
PaulaMediaandEntertainment.com, Nashua, NH
ISBN: 9781542726054
Edition Notice
Date of Publication: December 21, 2016
Number of Printings: First printing
Year of publication: 2016

Books may be purchased by contacting the publisher and author at:
Books may be purchased in quantity and/or special sales by contacting
the publisher, PaulaMediaandEntertainment.com or by email at
Frably@aol.com.

Books may be purchased in quantity and/or special sales by contacting
the publisher,

Library of Congress Catalog Number:
ISBN:
  1. Infertility 2. Fertility 3. Health

     First Edition

Paula Fuoco Davis: is a journalist and life coach. She has been a a writer since she was in fourth grade and her beloved teacher Mrs. Klein knelt down and told her 'you could be a writer' after writing an essay about water. For more than 30 years, she worked as a newspaper reporter and journalist for The Lawrence Eagle-Tribune, The Nashua Telegraph and New Hampshire magazine. She covered education, social issues and features. She founded and is editor of Commitment.com, an online site for women and authored more than 25 books. She is a survivor of infertility and wants others to have every single bit of information she didn't have. She has loved writing this book.

Yes, I Can Get Pregnant: Letters For Infertility Patients To Send Themselves

During your fertility journey, there are times you will need to be your own best friend. Here are letters that you can mail to yourself, or just leave around the house when you need a lift or a reminder of how strong you are.

Be sure to begin each letter by filling in your name and then signing it at the end. Read the letters aloud. Tuck them in your purse and read throughout the day. Tape them to a mirror, hang them on a wall, or put them on the refrigerator.

Dear_____,

Congratulations! You are on your way to getting pregnant! Today, you are close to being pregnant!

Every day, your body is getting stronger. I see you getting stronger!

You are ready and your body is to conceive a baby.

You are ready to have a baby! That's right--your body can easily conceive a baby now! Congratulations!

Love,

_____

Dear _____,

I know with all my heart that you will give birth to a baby soon.

Yes, you, are capable of giving birth soon.

Your dear sweet ovaries, your healthy healthy ovaries, can produce ripe, rich healthy eggs.

Actually, right now you are making healthy fertile eggs!

Your ovaries know how to produce good eggs.

Your ovaries are right now producing eggs that will lovingly grow into your baby.

Thank you ovaries! Thank you for giving me healthy fertile eggs that will grow within me and enable me to conceive my baby!

Love,

_____

Dear _____,

You are ready to be a mother. I can see it—you are ready.

Nothing in your past can hold you back from having a child.

You deserve to give birth! You are worthy of this!

There is nothing for you to fear when it comes to becoming a mother.

You can do this.

Millions of women from various backgrounds, life experiences and families give birth and raise children. So can you.

You do not need to be perfect to be a good mother. Go ahead, let yourself have this. You deserve a baby.

Love,

_____

Dear _____,

Your vagina, your dear beautiful healthy vagina, is ready to receive.

Yes, vagina, you are ready to receive. Thank you for welcoming my baby.

Thank you vagina for opening up and allowing, welcoming and helping my baby in.

Thank you vagina for being a safe place for my baby.

I love you vagina. I love everything about you. Thank you for receiving my child and giving it a safe home to grow.

Love,

_____

Dear _____,

I think you know this, but I will say it again: it is safe for you to have a baby.

It is safe for you to get pregnant.

It is safe for you to carry a child for nine months.

It is safe for you to give birth. It is safe for you to be a mother.

Love,

_____

Dear _____,

Hi! I'm writing to let you know that yes, you are fertile and strong!

You are capable of having a baby soon!

You are fertile and strong!

All your organs and hormones are working together so you can conceive and give birth very, very soon!

I love you! I love you! I love you! All the organs in your body love you! They want to help you! All your hormones love you! They want to help you!

I love you and know you are going to give birth soon.

Love,

_____

Dear_____,

You, my darling, are a part of the world's unstoppable, undefeatable, always victorious life and birth cycle.

You are an important part of the birth cycle that goes on around you each day.

See that flower blooming: you are part of that bloom.

See that baby squirrel: you are part of the natural birth cycle that goes on in the world.

You are an integral part of all the birth and life that goes on around you each day.

You are part of life's most beautiful and welcoming birth cycle.

You have everything you need within you to give birth to a baby, just like all the other living beings on this planet. You've got it kid! You do!

You are part of the birth cycle of life that permeates the world.

Congratulations!

Love,

_____

Dear _____,

Your liver is healthy and clean. Your liver has released all the anger within it. Your liver is working hard to release the toxins within you.

Amazing liver, I love everything you are doing to help me get pregnant. I love you liver!

I love everything about you!

Liver, you are calm and happy now. You have released all anger.

Liver, you are doing a fine job of helping me get pregnant.

Thank you, my strong and happy liver, for helping me make my baby.

Love,

_____

Dear_____,

Hello beautiful kidneys! I love you kidneys!

I thank you kidneys for releasing all the sadness that used to be in me.

You, my sweet kidneys, are filled with happiness now. You, strong and beautiful kidneys, give off happy, healthy energy now!

Thank you kidneys, for allowing yourself to be filled with joy, peace and hope, and that you are sharing that with me, so I can get pregnant soon.

I love you kidneys. I love everything about you. Thank you kidneys for helping me get pregnant. Thank you for releasing all fear and shame, and being the healthy strong kidneys I know you can be.

Love,

_____

Dear _____,

Congratulations! Your dream of being a mother is about to come true!

Love,

_____

Dear _____,

I give you permission to get pregnant.

I give you permission to conceive.

You have permission to be pregnant.

You have permission to conceive.

It is right and good for you to have a baby.

You are allowed to have a baby.

Permission to have a baby is yours.

Love,

_____

Dear _____,

Hello adrenal glands! You are full of abundant, brilliant, vibrant energy!

Adrenal glands, you are balanced and calm.

Adrenal glands, you are full of healthy, beautiful energy.

Your adrenal glands are full of energy.

I thank you adrenals for being so full of good, strong energy.

Adrenal glands, thank you for helping me have a baby. Thank you for your energy and your love.

Thank you, adrenals, for giving me what I need to have my baby.

Thank you for being powerful and full of good energy. I love you adrenals so much.

Love,

_____

Dear _____,

You are good enough right now in this moment to have a baby.

You are healthy enough in this moment to have a baby!

You are strong enough in this moment to have a baby!

You are worthy and deserving in this moment to have a baby!

You have everything within you in this moment to conceive and give birth to a baby!

Love,

_____

Dear _____,

Today, your life is filled with joy.

Today, your life is good and good things like a baby growing within you are flowing to you naturally.

You are happy. Your heart is happy. Your body is happy.

Your body is happy because it knows you are going to have a baby soon.

Your body is happy because it is going to help you have a baby soon.

Your body is ready and able to help you conceive and give birth.

Wow, life is so good right now. Everything is so good right now. Joy fills your heart and all your organs—you are happy, happy, happy!

Today that happiness is you!!!

Today your body is saying that it can conceive and it can give birth!!!

Love,

_____

Dear _____,

Stop being scared. It is safe for you to be a mother.

It is good for you to be a mother.

There is only good that will come from your experience of being a mother.

It is safe for you to be a mother.

It is safe for you to give birth to a baby.

It is safe for you to be pregnant.

It is safe to receive a baby.

Having a baby is safe for you.

Love,

_____

Dear _____,

Guess what? Your hormones are balanced and your reproductive system is working well.

Guess what? Your body is able to receive and conceive.

Congratulations!

Love,

_____

Dear _____,

You are capable of enjoying a healthy pregnancy.

You are very capable of carrying your baby full-term.

Your body knows how to hold and care for your baby for nine months.

Your body knows how to give birth.

Your body knows how to stay balanced and give your growing baby everything is needs to be born healthy and strong.

Your body has everything it needs to conceive and carry your baby for nine healthy and happy months—and then it knows how to deliver and give birth to your baby too! Congratulations!

Love,

_____

Dear _____,

Thank you, my beautiful body, for helping me heal from infertility.

Thank you for being my friend and helping me to have the baby of my dreams.

Thank you ovaries for producing ripe, healthy, fertile eggs.

Thank you liver and ovaries, for managing my hormones with love and care, so that everything is flowing and balanced as it should be.

Thank you adrenals for being so calm and balanced and full of vibrant energy.

Thank you thyroid for being so calm and balanced and able to do your job well.

Thank you body, for everything you are doing to make sure I get pregnant soon! I love you and appreciate all you do.

Love,

_____

Dear _____,

You are worthy of having a baby!

You are full of pure brilliant energy that has healed you from infertility.

You are full of love for your future babies.

You are full of smiles and happiness and joy that has healed you!

Love,

_____

Dear _____,

Things can work out for you.
Things will work out for you.
Things can go right for you.
Things will go right for you.

Love,

_____

Dear _____,

I love everything about you! I love you kidneys! I love you liver! I love you hormones! I love you adrenal glands! I love you thyroid! I love you ovaries! I love you vagina!

I love your energy! I love your strength! I love that you are about to conceive your baby! I love that you will be giving birth soon!

Love,

_____

Dear _____,

All trauma and sadness has left your body. Love has entered your organs and cells instead.

Goodbye sadness! Goodbye sad memories from the past! Goodbye trauma!

Love is pouring in your body now.

Love lives everywhere in your body.

Loving memories…loving thoughts…loving ideas…loving people…loving lives inside you.

All difficulties from your childhood have left. Goodbye sad memories! Love is pouring in its place. Hello love!

Now, there is no trauma left in your body. There is nothing sad in your body. There is nothing scared in your body. All fear has left. All sadness has left.

Only love remains. Only love flows through your body.

Only joy and happiness and giggles and smiles live in your body.

Go ahead, smile. Smile! Everything is good! I can see so much love flowing through your body.

There is no more trauma, no more bad memories, no more worries.

Your body has let go! The sadness is gone. The trauma is gone. Love is here and soon your baby will be here too!

Love,

Dear _____,

All your hormones are in balance.

All your hormones communicate well with one another and work together in the most loving way possible.

All your hormones are friends and they have all agreed to help you get pregnant.

Your hormones are balanced and calm, full of beautiful flowing energy.

Your hormones understand their job and do their job well.

Your hormones know how to give you what you need to get pregnant.

Your hormones know how to give your body what it needs to stay pregnant.

Your hormones know how to help your body give birth.

Love,

_____

Dear _____,

Your kidneys are running perfectly. Your adrenals are filled with energy. Your ovaries are in perfect balance producing perfect eggs. Your uterine is open and welcoming.

Every part of your body is in sync.

Every part of your body is filled with love.

Every part of your body is running exactly and perfectly as it should be.

Every part of your body is doing exactly what it needs to do to conceive and help you get pregnant.

Love,

_____

Dear _____,

You have all the help you need to get pregnant.

You have all the help you need to stay pregnant for nine months and give birth.

Everyone is here to help you.

We are all here to help you.

You are surrounded by help.

You have all the help you need.

Love,

_____

Dear _____,

Go ahead and have a baby! Its okay! You've got permission!

Love,

_____

Dear _____,

I am here for you. You are not alone. I love you. I will help you. I will take care of you. I will help you every step of the way!

I love you. I am here for you. Don't be scared—together we can do this!

You are not alone.

We will conceive this baby together. We will carry this baby together.

We will give birth together. You are not alone. You are not left to do this yourself. You have help. You have me.

Love,

_____

Dear _____,

Your body just told me it wants to be pregnant.

Your body just told me that it knows how to get pregnant.

Your body just told me that it is going to get pregnant.

You are fertile! You are ripe and fertile! Your body just told me so.

Love,

_____

Dear _____,

We all love you. We all believe you can do this.

We all believe you can conceive a baby, carry it for nine months safely, and give birth beautifully.

Don't be scared. Together, we can do this.

Love,

_____

Dear _____,

Your desire to have a baby makes you powerful.

Your desire to be a mother makes you strong.

Your love for children makes you very, very fertile.

Your desire to give birth makes you successful.

Your yearning to be a mother makes you capable of conceiving.

Your desire to have a baby enables your body to give you what you want.

You are able, capable, and ready to conceive a baby.

You are ready to give birth.

You are ready to be a mother.

Love,

_____

Dear _____,

There is no reason why you can't have a baby. NO REASON!

There is nothing that can stop you from having a baby. NOTHING!

Don't be afraid. You can do this. Go ahead now—go have a baby!

Love,

_____

Dear _____,

Everyone thinks you will be a great mother.

Everyone thinks you are good enough to be a mother.

Everyone thinks you are strong enough to give birth.

I think you are ready to be pregnant.

I think being a mother is right for you.

I think having a baby is going to happen soon for you.

Love,

_____

Dear _____,

Adrenal glands, you are strong and working well.
Liver, you are strong and working well.
Hormones, you are balanced and working well.
Kidneys, you are strong and working well.
Thyroid, you are strong and working well.
Ovaries, you are strong and working well.
Fallopian tubes, you are strong and working well.

All the parts of your body are strong and working well.

Love,

_____

Dear _____,

You are full of courage. All fear has left your body.

You now can move forward with your dreams.

You are not stuck. You are flowing with courage and joy.

You are peaceful. You are filled with love. You are happy.

Your body is full of happiness. Sadness and grief has left your body.

Goodbye grief! Goodbye sad memories from the past!

Joy is pouring into your body instead.

Frustration is leaving your body. All frustration has left your body.

You are filled with power instead.

All your happiness and power is helping you to get pregnant.

You will be pregnant soon. You will enjoy a safe, healthy pregnancy. You will give birth soon.

Love,

_____

Dear _____,

All the parts of your body are ready to conceive a child.

All the parts of your body want you to know that they love you and are ready to help you give birth to a child.

Your liver, ovaries, adrenal glands, thyroid, and vagina, are all in agreement that they can help you make a baby.

They love you. They want you to know they love you very much, and they will help you conceive and give birth to a baby.

Love,

_____

Dear _____,

You are not going to repeat the mistakes your parents made when you were growing up.

I repeat: you are not going to repeat the mistakes your parents made growing up.

You are aware and you know how to learn from the mistakes of others.

You don't have to be perfect to perfectly and lovingly raise a child.

You will raise your child in safety and love. You will not repeat the past.

Love,

_____

Dear _____,

Trust that your body can give you a baby.

Trust that your body is now healing from infertility.

Trust that everything can work out for you.

Trust that your body knows how to conceive and enjoy a healthy pregnancy.

Trust that your body and heart know how to make a baby.

Trust that love surrounds you and your future babies.

Trust that your body can make a baby right now.

Love,

_____

Dear _____,

I give you permission to have a baby.

Yes, you have permission to have a baby.

You have permission to have as many babies as you want.

Love,

_____

Dear _____,

I grant you the power to have a baby.

You now can grant yourself the power to have a baby.

The power to conceive and give birth is already within you.

You can allow yourself to get pregnant.

You can freely and confidently allow yourself to become a mother.

The power to have a baby is already yours.

Your body is a healthy and perfect place for your baby to grow.

Relax and feel confident in the power within you.

Love,

_____

Dear_____,

Your mind, heart and body is a nourishing place for your future babies.

Your womb is strong and fertile.

Your uterus is a loving place to grow.

Accept the miracle of birth that is coming into your life.

You are part of the natural birth cycle.

It is safe for your baby to be born.

Your body, mind and heart all agree they are ready for you to give birth.

You are healthy and ready to conceive.

You are able to carry a pregnancy full-term and give birth to a healthy baby.

Let it happen.

Love,

_____,

Dear _____,

Don't be afraid to have a baby.

There is nothing to fear.

Love,

_____

Dear _____,

You have nothing to be ashamed of.

All shame must leave your body right now.

You deserve to feel confident, happy and joyful.

Anyone who ever shamed you must now exit the room.

Any experience that ever left you feeling ashamed will now dissolve and disappear.

Shame has left you.

Confidence has entered.

Love,

_____

Dear _____,

It is good to be a woman.

Everything female about you is something to be proud of.

It is good to be a woman.

Being female is good.

I love everything feminine about you.

Love,

_____

Dear _____,

If there is something in your past that is holding you back from having a baby, it now has no hold over you.

Anything negative in the past that is hurting your fertility must now disappear.

Its power over you is gone.

Its power to hurt you is erased.

The past cannot damage your fertility any longer.

You are fertile and strong and nothing can stop that.

You are fertile! Your reproductive organs are working well! The past has no hold over your body any longer.

Your body is running free and happy. It can do what it wants to do!

Your body wants to have a baby and nothing can stop it!

Your body is free! Let it be free to do what it wants to do!

Yay! You have survived and now are thriving!

Love,

_____

Dear _____,

It is okay to be authentically who you really are.

Stop hiding.

Stop being someone you are not.

Stop hiding your light.

Stop being afraid.

Stop denying yourself. Stop being who others tell you to be.

Stop being ashamed of your feelings. Stop feeling ashamed of things in your past.

Stop letting 'it' define you in a negative way.

Who you are is a beautiful woman who wants to conceive a baby and give birth.

Let yourself be who you want to be. Let your body do what it wants to do.

Shake off the shame. Let go of the tightness within you. Be you as much as possible.

Welcome every part of who you are back! You were always enough! Let yourself blossom as you were always suppose to blossom! There she is! Let her be! Let her be herself! She deserves that! She always did!

Trust her. Love her. Accept her. Let her do what she wants. Let her be herself. Stop trying to control and deny her.

She will feel better and so will you.

Love,

Dear_____,

Your true self is ready to be reunited with you.

Your true self flows naturally in your body.

Your true self feels comfortable and at home in her body.

Let all the energy, nourishment and peace within you flow.

Let her know she is valued and accepted.

Let her know she can be real and having a baby is something real she knows how to do.

Give yourself the freedom to be yourself.

Let your heart sing. You are allowed to be happy. You are allowed to have what you want. You are allowed to breath!

Breath! Give her what she wants! Breath! Let what is natural happen within you.

Let your body flow naturally as it wants to flow.

Love,

_____

Bonus: A Personal Fertility Vision Statement

Excerpted from Dancing Your Way to Fertility, available on Amazon.com

It is a bright, warm, sunny morning and you are feeling really good. You walk outside, take a deep breath of fresh air, raise your arms to the sky and say thank you, thank you, thank you for my baby.

That's right, YOUR NAME_____, having a baby is easy for you. Your body and mind are ready, willing and VERY able to have a baby.

You smile, because being vibrantly healthy and super fertile feels good.

Really good actually.

You know on a very deep level that having a baby is good and right for you. You deserve this baby. You are completely and totally worthy of having a baby. You are capable of conceiving a baby, carrying a baby for nine months and giving birth, in the healthiest, safest, most wonderful way possible.

That's right, you are worthy of having children.

Because you ate so many healthy green vegetables, let go of the toxins in your body, and said goodbye to all the trauma, anger and sadness in your cells, you are now able to give birth to a baby whenever you choose.

That's right: you can have a baby whenever you want to. Today, next week, next month, whenever you choose. Your body has the power to conceive and give birth to a baby whenever you want it to.

You can see yourself smiling and holding your new baby. You see yourself kissing your baby and feeling so thankful that your baby has arrived.

You look in the mirror and smile, because being a mother feels right to you.

Your baby is here. You are fertile. You are super fertile today! You are actually over-the-top fertile right now! You are creating super healthy eggs this minute.

That's right: your dear sweet ovaries are right now producing ripe, rich, healthy eggs. Feel how strong and good your eggs are!

Your body now has everything it needs to get pregnant. All the organs in your body are working at maximum capacity to help you get pregnant. Your liver has let go of anger and is now balanced and calm. Your kidneys have let go of sadness and are happy now.

Nothing in your past can block you from conceiving and giving birth. You forgive those who hurt you. You released all anger and sadness. You have let go of all the bad memories, sad events, and traumas in your life. Only happiness lives in your cells now.

Love and happiness flow through your body now. Love flows into your heart.

That's right, there is immense power in your heart to have a baby.

You have permission to have a baby. You have permission to conceive. You have permission to enjoy a safe and successful pregnancy. You are ready to give birth.

Your hurt is gone. Your anger is gone. Your fear is gone. You are safe.

That's right, you feel safe all the time. Safer than you ever felt before. You know it is safe for you to get pregnant and safe for you to give birth and safe for you to be a mother. Life is safe. Motherhood is safe. Having children is safe. Everything is safe.

You feel safe all the time, because you know that having a baby is safe for you.

All fears and pain from your childhood are gone. All your anxiety is gone. All your frustration is gone.

You laugh and feel happy.

That's right, you laugh a lot lately, because feeling so healthy and fertile feels good.

Really good actually. Life is so good!

Your body is now full of pure and clean energy. Your bowels are clean and you eliminate easily. Your blood sugar levels are stable. Your hormones are balanced and communicate well with one another. Your pituitary gland, adrenal gland, thyroid and pancreas are healthy and balanced. Blood flows easily to your uterus. Oxygen flows easily to your ovaries. Your uterine lining is strong. Your vagina is open and ready to receive. Your ovaries are making lots of healthy eggs.

That's right, your ovaries are now making strong, viable healthy eggs that make it easy for you to conceive and give birth.

You now flow with life. You feel comfortable asserting your will. You let your authentic voice be heard. You welcome your real self. You respect yourself. You no longer feel shame or guilt. You honor and express all your feelings. You creativity express yourself, as having a baby is a creative expression you fully allow yourself.

You smile and feel relaxed.

You feel relaxed a lot lately. You slept so good last night. You sleep good every night.

That's right, you are relaxed and sleeping well because you know everything is going to be okay.

It is okay for you to get pregnant and have lots of babies.

You smile, because you always knew you would get pregnant.

That's right. You knew that infertility was just a temporary condition. You knew you would heal and be fertile. You always said, "I will get pregnant soon" and you were right.

You have already let yourself receive a baby. Your womb is a warm, welcoming place for your babies.

You are strong enough to receive and hold your baby.

Nothing in your past can hold you back having the children you desire. You deserve this! Go ahead. Let yourself have this. Let yourself have your babies!

You, my darling, are part of the world's unstoppable, undefeatable, always victorious birth cycle. See that flower blooming—you are part of that bloom. See that tree sprouting new leaves—you are part of that sprouting! You are part of life's beautiful birth cycle. You have everything you need within you to give birth to a baby, just like all the other living beings on the planet.

You got it kid! You do! Your dream of being a mother is now coming true. You are allowed to have a baby. It is good and right and okay for you to have a baby. It is safe for you to be a mother.

That's right—you are meant to have a baby. Things are working out for you, just as you hoped they would.

It feels right and good to receive your baby. Your body feels good doing this. Giving birth is fun. Being a mother is fun. Getting pregnant is fun.

Go ahead and have a baby! It is okay! You have given yourself permission! Every part of your body has agreed to help you conceive and give birth.

Getting pregnant is easy for you.

Go ahead, today is the day you can conceive your beautiful baby.

Then do it again whenever you want too, because getting pregnant and having children is easy, safe and fun for someone like you.

A Bonus Excerpt from Dancing Your Way to Fertility available on Amazon.com and at <u>www.dancingyourwaytofertility.com</u>.

Infertility: A Training Ground for Motherhood?

In times past, women have always endured sacrifice and trial as part of motherhood. Now, due to a host of factors such as age, health and environment, women are put through a severe test of their maternal stamina even before they conceive their child.

This road, this test, this initiation, will test all of you--and it will make you one of the strongest, most capable, confident, resourceful, perseverant mothers a child could ever have. Experiencing infertility gives you a lifetime pass to enjoy motherhood in a way few ever get to enjoy it, because with the difficulties of this disease come confidence and appreciation.

This journey will demand all the best parts of you. It will demand you persevere when you want to give up.

It will demand patience and persistence when frustration and helpless surrender might feel like a more natural path.
It will demand that every survival skill you possess be brought forth and utilized. It will demand sacrifice, self-preservation, and a willpower beyond what you knew you had, but what intrinsically you knew you were capable of.

If you are not fortunate, you may have your heart broken in 1000 pieces.

If you are fortunate, you could still have your heart broken in 1000 places.

When you give birth to your baby none of it will matter. Your heart will heal, the scars will seem insignificant, and all the tears, disappointments and devastations will seem like bunny rabbits and balloons on a summer's day.

No big deal.

If you do not give birth to a baby, but decide to adopt, become a foster parent, a teacher, coach, counselor or play a very active role in the life of a young niece, nephew, neighbor, or cousin, you will be ready and able to mother these children and impact a younger generation in a way more powerful than you ever imagined.

You have probably been through the best training course for motherhood possible: you understand pain, you understand the potential for joy, you are willing to do the work to get the child you want, and you've proven you can take the bad stuff that comes with going after the good stuff. In doing this, you will join a group of super cultivated mothers, women ready to nurture and love the next generation, and have more than proven their worth to do this.

Infertility hurts.

Winning over infertility can be a painful process that demands resolve and sacrifice.

It is an initiation rite, of sorts, an involuntary one, of course.

No one should have to go through this to have a baby and no one would voluntarily choose this road. Nonetheless, it is a reality for many of us, and it will prepare you for motherhood in a grand and inspiring way that someday you may even feel thankful to have experienced.

It is a long road and an unfair one, but at the end of the road, you could be holding the baby of your dreams, just as the same as someone who made love one night and woke up pregnant the next morning.

Then nothing at all will matter but your baby.

12 Cleanses To Help Restore Your Fertility

A Bonus Excerpt from Dancing Your Way to Fertility available on Amazon.com and at <u>www.dancingyourwaytofertility.com</u>.

The next step in changing the state, or condition, of your body is cleansing and detoxifying. The importance of detoxifying your body should never be underestimated. In this chapter, we'll look at 12 cleanses that can help restore and maximize your fertility potential.

Please note: cleanses should be done before you start infertility medications or treatments, because you do not want them to interfere with medications or a pregnancy, if there is even a slight chance you could be pregnant. Cleansing can be compared to overturning and fertilizing the soil before planting the seed.

If you are just starting infertility treatments, you may want to choose just one or two cleanses, so as not to delay treatment.

If you've been trying to get pregnant for a long time with no success, you might want to consider doing various cleanses to strengthen your body.
Here are some cleanses to consider:

• A Liver Cleanse

Never never NEVER underestimate the importance of having your liver cleaned and detoxified. The liver is a highly influential organ that plays a key role in fertility and is one of the most important organs in your body.

The liver governs approximately 500 metabolic processes and many studies have shown that the oestrogen receptors in the liver are critical for maintaining fertility.

I cannot say enough about the importance of having a clean, de-toxified liver in the quest to get pregnant.

An ineffective liver allows toxins to seep into the ovaries and endocrine system.

If your liver is congested, it cannot adequately remove toxins and fats from the body.

Instead, they will continue to recirculate through your system—causing hormonal disturbances and imbalances. It also means your ovaries will be flooded with toxic substances that your liver was suppose to clean—and your ovaries are the source of your eggs. These impurities will result in poor egg quality—all because your liver was too congested to do its job. So if you want to improve the quality of your eggs, make sure your liver is as clean and detoxified as possible.

Once the liver is cleansed, the entire endocrine and reproductive system becomes free of toxins and impurities, so they can begin functioning at a higher capacity.

What causes a sluggish, tired liver? Stress, poor diet, medication, toxins in the environment, low-quality food, coffee, sugar, white flour products and low quality drinking water, are among a few of the culprits. The older we get, the more our liver needs to be cleaned out because of the junk that we have taken into our body over the years.

A liver cleanse will help kick your body into high gear, increasing energy and vitality to all your organs.

Liver cleanses can be found online and at most health and natural food stores.

You may want to do a 30-day cleanse more than once. Please note: A liver cleanse should never be done while you are taking infertility medications, as it could interfere with the effectiveness of the medication. It is something to do BEFORE you begin any infertility treatments or medication, and is never to be done if you could be pregnant.

In addition to a liver cleanse, here are some other ways to detoxify, cleanse and strengthen your liver:

• Milk thistle is a wonderful herb for cleansing the liver. Read the directions on the bottle carefully as to amounts taken.

• Lemon is a great liver cleanser. About 20 minutes before breakfast in the morning, squeeze the juice from one or two fresh lemons into some warm water and drink.

• Beets are excellent liver cleansers. You can eat them cooked or juice them. To juice beets, peel and cut into small wedges that can easily fit in your juicer. Juice the beets with some apple, spinach or kale.

• Chlorophyll is a highly esteemed liver cleanser.

• Artichokes are powerful liver protectors because they contain a flavonoid called silymarin, which is an antioxidant that protects the liver from toxicity.

• Foods that are good for your liver include: spirulina, garlic, carrots, romaine lettuce, apples, grapefruit, chicory, mustard greens, dandelion greens, avocados, walnuts, turmeric and parsley.

• Cabbage can also be juiced and is effective in cleaning the liver.

• Amino acids, derived from healthy sources of protein, are key to the liver working at maximum capacity. Foods that contain these amino acids include: nuts, such as pumpkin seeds, squash seeds and almonds; lean meats, eggs, and beans, such as lentils and garbanzo.

• In Chinese medicine, infertility is often linked to Liver chi stagnation, a result of stress, overwork, and the effects of coffee and alcohol. Irritability, headaches and frustration are just some of the physical and emotional symptoms of liver chi stagnation. Acupuncturists and herbalists can work on unblocking energy stagnation in the liver.

• According to Chinese medicine, emotional and lifestyle cures for liver stagnation include being assertive, making clear decisions and enjoying lots of fun, laughter and relaxation. Holding on to anger, feeling stuck and depression impair the liver by stagnating the energy.

Letting go, moving on, and exercising control over one's life, can help in healing the liver.

For more cleanses, visit DancingYourWayToFertility.com or Amazon.com.

How to Improve Your Egg Quality

A Bonus Excerpt from Dancing Your Way to Fertility available on Amazon.com and at <u>www.dancingyourwaytofertility.com</u>.

Good news—you can improve the health and quality of your eggs.

In the past, we were told we were all born with a certain number of egg cells that run out as we age. We were led to believe that egg cells were the only cells in the body that did not regenerate, but instead were a finite number. We are finding out THIS IS JUST NOT TRUE. Recent research has shown that women can produce new eggs throughout their reproductive years.

You may have been told that your eggs are not healthy or that your eggs are too old.

Here's the great news: there is much you can do to enhance the health of your eggs.

It was commonly believed that the only factor that determined egg health and quality was age. Several new studies have shown that stress, hormones and environmental toxins all impact our egg health.

Your egg's health is a key cornerstone of a healthy fertility, because the health of your eggs can affect whether or not fertilization, implantation and ultimately a healthy pregnancy and birth will occur.

Here are some things you can do to improve your egg health:

• Coenzyme Q10: Coenzyme Q10 is an excellent way to improve the quality and energy within your eggs.

In several studies, the supplement Coenzyme Q10 has been shown to improve egg quality.

It boosts energy production in the oocytes, which are cells in the ovary. Providing additional energy in the form of Coenzyme Q10 is needed when there is decreased energy production in the ovaries due to aging.

It is also a source of fuel for the mitochondria, which produces energy within the cells and with age, can begin to weaken. Along with taking a Coenzyme Q10 supplement, natural sources of CoQ10 include almonds, spinach, sardines, broccoli, strawberries, and walnuts.

For more on egg health, Dancing Your Way to Fertility is available on Amazon.com or visit www.dancingyourwaytofertility.com.

The People In Your Journey and Some of the Rude Comments You May Hear Along the Way

A Bonus Excerpt from Dancing Your Way to Fertility available on Amazon.com and at www.dancingyourwaytofertility.com.

This is not to be misinterpreted as an exercise in dumping family or friends, because people are not perfect and we should not expect them to be, and there are people in our lives, as unpleasant as they may be, that we simply need to forgive, stay connected to and be around.

Despite their flaws, we owe them something. That being said, as you walk this journey, you need to be ready for some of the stupid, rude and totally insensitive comments you are going to hear. Sometimes, people you love will say really dumb things.

Other times, it could be a stranger who zaps you with a statement that leaves you breathless and feeling punched in the gut.

Here are a few of the stupid, rude, thoughtless and COMPLETELY FALSE comments you may have to deal with, and how best to respond:

• **"Maybe you weren't meant to have a baby":** Yes, you were meant to have a baby. Yes, you were.

Millions of women have babies whether they want them or not, whether they will be good mothers or not, so why shouldn't you have a baby? In fact, there is NOT ONE REASON IN THIS UNIVERSE why you should not have a baby.

This person is either jealous of you or just likes to pop the balloon of hope. People who mouth off a comment like this mistakenly feel they have some sort of moral authority. Ignore them. They are wrong. Completely and utterly wrong.

• **"Aren't you a little too old to be trying for a baby?"**

Whoever got the idea that a young mother is better than an older mother has not seen the millions of mothers in their 40s and even 50s who mother with great patience, love, insight, wisdom and kindness.

This person obviously doesn't understand that with age comes maturity and wisdom.

Someone who makes a comment like this may be focusing on the energy level of children, forgetting that even most 25 year old mothers are not out playing baseball with their kids everyday.

Whoever throws out a comment about age is ignorant of the fact that a woman of any age who is ready and able to love a child, and who is brave and strong enough to endure infertility, is more prepared, capable and ready to mother than almost anyone. A good mother is a good mother, whether she is 21, 31, 41, 51 or beyond.

Letting Go Of the Secret Thoughts and Hidden Beliefs That Might be Holding You Back from Getting Pregnant

A Bonus Excerpt from Dancing Your Way to Fertility available on Amazon.com and at <u>www.dancingyourwaytofertility.com</u>.

You may find this hard to believe, but hidden within your subconscious could be some negative perceptions of pregnancy, childbirth and motherhood that are holding you back from having a baby, without you even knowing it.

You may have some hidden fears or beliefs about becoming a mother that conflict with your desire to have a baby.

Sometimes, the body can hold two very different desires at once. One part of us wants one thing, another part of us wants another.

Consciously, you may want to become a mother more than anything in the world. Subconsciously, you may have fears that are making it hard for your conscious wishes to come true. These two very different parts of you could be playing a tug of war: who will win? Who will get their way? Whose needs will be met? This conflict can make it hard for us to really commit and do the work needed to get what we want.

This tug of war steals energy away from what your body really needs to be doing—and that is healing and getting pregnant.

Ultimately, the goal should be that all the different parts of you are working harmoniously together and have the same goal: to conceive a baby.

Deep fears and childhood issues sometimes need to be acknowledged, listened to and healed so you can move forward in having a child.

It is important that you discover and acknowledge all your feelings and beliefs about becoming a mother—even the ones that are not all warm and fuzzy. Our conscious self might want something, but if our subconscious does not want it, it could be off doing a dance of its own.

If your subconscious doesn't want something, your body could follow suit.

Subconscious fears about pregnancy, child birth or raising a child could even at times influence your hormones and the physical processes required for conception.

Does having doubt, fear, or hesitance about having children mean you won't be a great mother? Not at all. Millions of great Moms once had doubts or fears about becoming a mother. Millions more worried about pregnancy, childbirth and how their life would change. Embarking on a new life path naturally brings up feelings of doubt and fear.

To find out what your subconscious really thinks about getting having a child, start by asking yourself what you think about becoming a mother, and then write down whatever response comes from you without editing yourself. Allow your subconscious to voice its feelings on the subject without judgment or criticism.

Negative feelings or beliefs left unexpressed or unresolved hold considerable energy which can block conception. If you ignore your subconscious, it might stage a rebellion within your body—not allowing you to get pregnant because it wasn't given the respect and attention it deserved.

Begin by writing: "I will become pregnant soon" or "My womb is ready to receive" and then after you write that, start writing whatever comes up from deep within.

Let whatever comes up from within you come up, come out and be heard. Write without editing or judging what you are writing.

Do not consciously think about what is coming up, or try to force something you don't really feel or think. Just write.

This exercise can help you uncover what you are feeling about your infertility on many levels. It can also reveal if there is a part of you that wants to sabotage your efforts to become pregnant, or feels that you are not worthy of a baby. By knowing your innermost feelings, you can then work on bringing together the different emotions within you, so that you can achieve your goal. Later on, reread what you wrote and thank your subconscious for opening up.

Try not to judge your subconscious, even if what comes up is not exactly what you want to hear.

You could also write down the words: 'I deserve to have a baby' and then type or handwrite whatever comes up. Remember: No judging. No editing. No thinking this out. Write without restraint and let your deep internal self say what it needs to say.

Other writing prompts include:

• My body is ready to conceive and give birth to a baby
• It is safe to have a baby
• I deserve to have a baby
• I am good enough to be a mother and give birth to a baby
• My body is capable of giving birth
• A woman like me deserves to be a mother
• I am ready to be a mother and have children
• It is safe for me to become a mother
• Being a mother is a good thing for me

Honestly listening to every part of yourself shows your courage, because you are not going into denial.

Every part of you needs deserves to be listened to so they can all work together. If you ignore the needs of your subconscious, it could sabotage all the hard work you are doing to get pregnant.

Here are some questions to ask yourself, write responses to, and spend some time thinking about.

• **Are you afraid of repeating the same mistakes your parents made?:** Do you fear repeating some of the negative and dysfunctional family patterns you grew up with? Do you sometimes find yourself thinking, 'when I become a parent, I never want to do to my child what my parents did to me' or 'I never want to put my kids through what my parents put me through.'

• **Are you scared of becoming a mother?:** Do you have fears about becoming a mother, such as or 'I'm afraid of who I will become when I have a child' or 'I'm afraid I don't have what it takes to be a good Mom' or 'I'm afraid I won't be able to care for my child properly.'

• **Are you worried about losing some of your me-time once you have a baby?:** Are there aspects of your life that you really like that you are worried you will lose once you have a baby?

• **Do you fear that once you become a mother, you will turn into your own mother?:** Did your Mom behave or act in a way that you don't want to repeat and hurt you a lot as a child? Or did your Mom do things that you promised yourself you would never do? Did you long ago make a silent pact with yourself that you would never become your mother?

• **Do you sometimes feel infertility is a deserved punishment, either from yourself or from God, for something you've done or didn't do, in the past?:** Could infertility be something you think you deserve to suffer? Did you do something, or not do something, you believe merits you being infertile?

• **Do you feel God is mad at you?:** Do you feel God is judging you harshly for something you did in your past that you still feel guilty about?

• **Were you a victim of physical, sexual abuse or emotional abuse? Did you have an abusive parent?:** Do you ever fear that you will become an abusive parent like they were? If so, you might fear repeating negative family patterns.

• **Did you ever experience a trauma that has left you feeling unsafe and weary of new experiences?:** Are you open to new experiences or does doing something for the first time unnerve you? Do you often feel scared and worried about your safety?

A Bonus Excerpt from **The Infertility Diaries** available on Amazon.com and at www.dancingyourwaytofertility.com.

The Doctor Called My Eggs "Bottom of the Barrel"

My doctor looked at me point blank and said without a trace of mercy that my eggs were "bottom of the barrel."

Bottom of the barrel... Her words rang in my head like a cruel pronouncement.

I was 37 years old and desperately wanted a second child. My doctor didn't believe I could have one.

I had been through this before. To have my daughter, I endured 10 IUIs, several operations and too many nights of crying to count.

So I left her office: desperate, heartbroken, and wildly, frantically panicked. The words 'your eggs are bottom of the barrel' kept repeating in my head. Despite everything I've gone through, I always had hope. My insides were screaming: 'I can't live with this.' I was so shaken, I could barely drive home. Her words nearly broke my will and spirit to try again.

For some reason, on the way home, I stopped at a natural foods market. Walking around the supermarket, amidst all the healthy foods and supplements, I began to question what the doctor told me. Was the poor quality of my eggs something that could be improved? Was I unhealthy on some undetectable level that was impacting my fertility? I went home and called my ever-wise mother. She gave me great advice: dump that doctor and try again.

I did exactly what Mom said. I decided I would do everything I could to restore and heal my fertility, and not be hindered by my age, regardless of what the doctor said.

Over time, I learned that there was hope for me and others like me—and just because a doctor says you can never get pregnant does not mean your body, if given the right elements, cannot heal from infertility.

My devastation and despair turned to determination, and everything I learned, I put in this book. As a newspaper reporter for more than 25 years, I utilized my skills as a journalist to get to the root of fertility problems, the physical and the emotional.

I am now also a fertility success certified life coach and I wrote about how I healed my body in my book "Dancing Your Way to Fertility" that is also available on Amazon.com. That book includes my story, along with The Ultimate Fertility Success Program which I believe is one of the most comprehensive body-mind makeover plans available to fertility patients today.

The Ultimate Fertility Success Program includes 12 cleanses that will detoxify your body and expand your fertility potential.
It will also show you how to improve the quality of your eggs—something previously not thought possible—and balance your hormones.

In this book, The Infertility Diaries, I share my personal journey of battling infertility, a rotten opponent that needed to be knocked upside its head and kicked to the curb.

It wasn't easy and there were moments, as you will read, that nearly broke me.

That doctor who claimed my eggs were 'bottom of the barrel' was wrong. Less than a year later, I gave birth to my beautiful son.

Someday, I would like to send her a picture of my boy and write in blazing letters across the picture: "Is this what bottom of the barrel looks like?"

Very, Very Sad

It is June. One year and three months since I began infertility treatments. Such a long time and still no baby. I am sad. No, I am beyond sad--I am enraged, frustrated, full of yearning.

I am tired of yearning.

I long to hold hands with a baby...a baby that is mine.

I look at mothers in supermarkets, mothers who look angry, tired and annoyed at their rambunctious little brats and I think: God, why can't that be me? Why can't I be pushing around a cart full of loud, overtired, rambunctious children?

These mothers look so overworked, and yet they have no idea that I would do anything to have what they have.

These women look deceivingly ordinary in so many ways, and I think: why can't I have their ordinary life--the one that includes a grocery cart full of babies?

There is a woman I see occasionally who has four young children. She is beautiful and her children are lovely too.

When I saw her holding hands with one of her young sons the other day, I was struck with that image--the image of a woman holding hands with her son.

Hands to hold. I want little hands to hold.

When I see the little hands of a baby, I think: what in the world must it feel like to hold the little hands of a baby that you gave birth to? What I would give to hold such little hands, to know those hands were mine to hold, to know that those were the hands of my daughter or my son?

I am going to write Dr. P a letter to ask that he do a lapascropy to see if I have a problem with endometriosis.

I hope he listens and does what I want. I have to word the letter in a way that will get him to do as I ask.

I need little hands to hold. Hands that are all mine. To all the women I see shopping in supermarkets, who see themselves as ordinary mothers, I say--you have everything I want and there is nothing ordinary about your role as the mother to those little humans who are driving you crazy.

Please God, give me a little human to tire me out. Please let me be an ordinary mother in a supermarket one day.

I can't imagine anything in this world more special or more fun than pushing around my babies at the supermarket. My happy-ever-after is so plain and ordinary, boring even, and yet it feels so hopelessly impossible and faraway.

Meeting with Dr. P

I met with Dr. P today and found out a few disturbing things.

One is that yes, he knew I should be moving on to a stronger medicine, but because I tend to get scared and stressed during the procedures, he didn't think I could handle moving on to shots. I want to scream at him!

Instead, I force myself to stay calm and I explain to him that the more time that passes, the less nervous I am during procedures.

He seems skeptical, but I continue talking calmly, stating that while I may seem nervous, that is just my style of coping—and that the moment I leave the clinic, I feel completely calm and back to normal (which is true. I expulse everything and then I'm over it. It could be called being Italian, but I don't say that because it may sound weird.) He agrees to do the lapascropy and will schedule it soon. After that is done, depending on the outcome of the surgery, we will move on to shots. I am now waiting for a surgery date.

The Donut Incentive

They have ordered some new tests. This morning I was scheduled for a test I am dreading. I am so afraid of this particular test.

I don't think I have it in me to do this test. The whole drive down to the clinic, anxiety rattled around my body. How in the world am I going to make myself go through this test?

Then I got an idea: on the way to the clinic, I went to a drive-through Dunkin Donuts and ordered two of my favorite chocolate frosted donuts.

I get to the clinic, sit in the waiting room holding my donut bag, and soon am called in for the test. The nurse leaves the room while I change. When she comes back in, I am lying on the table, dressed in a johnny, with the donut bag sitting on my stomach.

"What are the donuts for?" she asks, straining to act like no-big-deal-so-what-if-a-bag-of-donuts-is-sitting-on-a-patient, but since she's not a professional actress, her irritation comes shining through.

"They are my reward for going through this test," I said.

My logic here is this: if I can lay here, endure whatever I have to endure, all the while seeing and smelling these two donuts that I am going to eat the moment the test is done, the test won't feel so bad or be so hard to take.

Nothing is a better reward for me than chocolate donuts.

The doctor comes in, and very politely asks if I want to eat the donuts sitting on my stomach before they do the test.

Again, he is trying to be nice, but obviously is a bit confused by the presence of the donut bag on my stomach.

The great efforts everyone went through to show respect to me, even though I obviously looked eccentric, was both hilarious and touching. What a nice group of people at this clinic.

"No," I giggled. "I'll eat them later," and it felt good to laugh and see the humor in this whole situation.

They did the test, and all the time I kept focusing on was: if I can get through this test, I can eat my donuts. I tried to think of nothing else, not the pain, not the nurses, not anything but the reward coming: the donuts. How I love chocolate donuts.

The test ended. Everyone left the room. Before I even changed out of the johnny, I devoured the donuts in about ten seconds.

Ah, the power of chocolate donuts.

Even the most unpleasant test was bearable because I had two grand and delicious donuts to look forward to. Maybe I'll try this again.

The Infertility Diaries is available at Amazon.com and at www.dancingyourwaytofertility.com.

www.ingramcontent.com/pod-product-compliance
Lightning Source LLC
Chambersburg PA
CBHW081410280526
45788CB00009B/3045